Enhancing Bust Elasticity: A Comprehensive Guide to Breast Fitness

Margaret Holden

Table of Contents

Chapter 1: Introduction

In the realm of beauty and wellness, the desire for optimal physical health and appearance is a shared aspiration. The focus of this comprehensive guide is on a specific aspect of well-being that holds significance for many individuals – bust elasticity. This introductory chapter sets the stage for our journey into understanding the importance of enhancing bust elasticity, exploring the underlying science, and discovering effective ways to achieve and maintain healthier, more resilient breasts.

The Significance of Bust Elasticity:

Breasts are not only a symbol of femininity but also play a vital role in physical and emotional well-being. Bust elasticity, the ability of breast tissue to stretch and rebound, is a key factor in maintaining the youthful appearance and functionality of the breasts. It influences aspects ranging from posture and comfort to body confidence and overall health. As such, understanding how to enhance and preserve bust elasticity is not just about aesthetics, but about promoting self-care and body positivity.

A Journey into the Science:

To truly grasp the concept of bust elasticity, we delve into the scientific underpinnings that shape breast health. We explore the intricate network of collagen and elastin fibers that contribute to the breasts' firmness, the hormonal influences that impact tissue structure, and the role of genetics in determining bust characteristics. By unraveling the science, we empower ourselves with knowledge to make informed decisions about our bust health.

Holistic Wellness and Bust Elasticity:

This guide takes a holistic approach to bust fitness, acknowledging the interconnectedness of physical, emotional, and lifestyle factors. It emphasizes the importance of nutrition, exercise, skincare, posture, and stress management in nurturing bust elasticity. By recognizing the various components that contribute to bust health, we gain a comprehensive toolkit for maintaining well-rounded well-being.

A Personalized Journey:

Every individual's body is unique, and there is no one-size-fits-all approach to enhancing bust elasticity. Throughout this guide, we will explore customizable exercises, dietary tips, and self-care practices that can be tailored to your specific needs and preferences. Whether you're looking to prevent sagging, reduce stretch marks, or simply promote a healthier bust, this guide aims to provide you with the tools and insights to embark on a personalized journey toward enhanced bust elasticity.

In the chapters that follow, we will delve deeper into the science, strategies, and practical advice that can empower you to proactively care for your bust health. From understanding the role of collagen to discovering effective exercises and skincare routines, our exploration will equip you with the knowledge and confidence to embark on your path toward optimal bust elasticity and overall well-being.

Chapter 2: The Science Behind Bust Elasticity

The beauty and functionality of the breasts are intricately linked to their underlying biological structures. In this chapter, we will delve into the scientific foundations of bust elasticity – the remarkable quality that allows breast tissue to stretch, adapt, and return to its original form. By understanding the physiological processes and factors that contribute to bust elasticity, we gain insights into how to support and enhance this essential aspect of breast health.

Collagen and Elastin: The Architects of Elasticity

At the heart of bust elasticity lies a dynamic duo of proteins: collagen and elastin. Collagen provides structural support to breast tissue, while elastin imparts resilience and flexibility. Together, they form a network of fibers that lend firmness and the ability to recoil to the breasts. We will explore how these proteins interact, and how their presence in the breast tissue contributes to the supple and resilient nature of the bust.

Hormones and Bust Health

Hormones play a pivotal role in shaping the breasts throughout various life stages. We'll uncover how hormones, such as estrogen and progesterone, influence breast development, size, and elasticity.

Hormonal fluctuations, which occur during puberty, menstruation, pregnancy, and menopause, can impact the composition and structure of breast tissue. By understanding these hormonal shifts, we can appreciate their effects on bust elasticity and explore strategies to optimize hormonal balance.

Genetics and Bust Characteristics

Our genetic makeup contributes significantly to the unique features of our breasts. Certain genes influence breast size, shape, and elasticity. We'll delve into the hereditary factors that determine bust characteristics and examine how genetics intersect with lifestyle choices and environmental influences. Understanding the genetic underpinnings of bust health empowers us to make informed decisions to support and maintain bust elasticity.

The Lifespan of Bust Elasticity

Bust elasticity is not a static quality but a dynamic characteristic that evolves over time. We'll explore how factors like aging, weight fluctuations, and pregnancy can impact the stretching and retracting capacity of breast tissue. As we gain insights into how the passage of time affects bust elasticity, we can explore proactive strategies to preserve and enhance it through various life stages.

The Interplay of Nutrition and Bust Health
Nutrition is a cornerstone of overall health, and its impact extends to bust elasticity. We'll discuss the nutrients essential for collagen and elastin production, as well as foods that promote tissue health and vitality. By understanding the role of

nutrition in supporting bust elasticity, we empower ourselves to make dietary choices that contribute to the long-term health of our breasts.

Harnessing Science for Bust Care

As we journey through the intricacies of the science behind bust elasticity, we gain a deeper appreciation for the complexity of breast tissue and its responsiveness to internal and external influences. Armed with this knowledge, we are better equipped to make informed lifestyle choices, engage in targeted exercises, and adopt skincare practices that nurture and enhance bust elasticity. This chapter serves as a foundation for the practical strategies we will explore in subsequent chapters, offering a science-based understanding of how to care for and promote the elasticity of your bust.

Chapter 3: Nutrition for Bust Health

In this chapter, we shift our focus to the vital role that nutrition plays in supporting and maintaining the health and elasticity of the bust. Just as a balanced diet contributes to overall well-being, specific nutrients and dietary choices can have a profound impact on the resilience, tone, and appearance of breast tissue. By understanding the key nutrients involved and making informed dietary decisions, we can proactively nurture our bust health from the inside out.

Essential Nutrients for Bust Elasticity

Certain nutrients are particularly crucial for maintaining the health of collagen and elastin fibers within the breast tissue. We'll explore the significance of nutrients like vitamin C, which aids in collagen production, and vitamin E, which acts as an antioxidant to protect tissues from damage. Minerals such as zinc and copper play integral roles in tissue repair and maintenance. By incorporating these essential nutrients into our diets, we can promote the elasticity and vitality of our bust.

Foods that Promote Collagen and Elastin Production

The saying "you are what you eat" holds true when it comes to supporting bust elasticity. We'll delve into foods that are rich in collagen-building nutrients, such as lean proteins (e.g., poultry, fish, beans) and vegetables (e.g., bell peppers, leafy greens). Antioxidant-rich foods, such as berries and nuts, also contribute to skin and tissue health. By choosing a diet abundant in these collagen-boosting foods, we can optimize the conditions for healthy breast tissue.

Hydration and its Effects on Bust Health

Staying adequately hydrated is often overlooked but is essential for maintaining the health of all bodily tissues, including breast tissue. We'll explore the role of water in promoting cellular health and maintaining skin elasticity. Dehydration can lead to dryness and reduced skin suppleness, potentially affecting the appearance and health of the bust. By prioritizing hydration, we support the overall health and vibrancy of our breasts.

Nutrition for Hormonal Balance

Hormonal fluctuations can impact bust health and elasticity. We'll discuss how certain nutrients, such as omega-3 fatty acids found in fatty fish, can help regulate hormonal levels and reduce inflammation. Balancing hormones through dietary choices can contribute to a more stable environment for breast tissue, positively affecting its elasticity and overall well-being.

Anti-Inflammatory Foods for Bust Health

Chronic inflammation can affect tissue health and elasticity. We'll explore the role of anti-inflammatory foods, such as turmeric, ginger, and green tea, in reducing inflammation and promoting overall bust health. By incorporating these foods into our diets, we can create an environment that supports the longevity and elasticity of breast tissue.

Creating a Nutrient-Rich Diet for Bust Health

Building a diet that promotes bust health requires a holistic approach. We'll provide guidance on creating well-rounded meals that incorporate a variety of nutrients necessary for optimal elasticity. By embracing a diverse range of nutrient-rich foods, we can maximize the benefits for our bust and overall health.

Long-Term Dietary Strategies for Bust Elasticity

Nutrition is a long-term investment in health, and the choices we make today can impact our well-being in the future. We'll discuss sustainable dietary strategies for maintaining bust elasticity over time. By adopting a balanced, nutrient-dense diet and making mindful dietary decisions, we can contribute to the lasting health and vitality of our bust.

As we explore the relationship between nutrition and bust health, we gain a deeper understanding of how our dietary choices influence the elasticity and appearance of our breasts. By incorporating these insights into our daily lives, we can harness the power of nutrition to support our quest for enhanced bust elasticity and overall well-being.

Chapter 4: Bust-Focused Exercises

In this chapter, we shift our attention to the physical aspect of enhancing bust elasticity through targeted exercises. Just as regular physical activity benefits overall health, specific exercises can help strengthen and tone the muscles that provide support to the bust area. By incorporating a variety of bust-focused exercises into your fitness routine, you can promote muscle engagement, posture improvement, and enhanced bust appearance.

Understanding the Bust Muscles

Before diving into the exercises, it's important to familiarize yourself with the muscles that contribute to bust support and appearance. We'll explore the pectoral muscles, which lie beneath the breasts and play a key role in maintaining breast firmness and lift. Understanding how these muscles function will provide context for the exercises that follow.

Effective Workouts for Bust Muscles

We'll delve into a range of exercises that specifically target the pectoral muscles. These exercises may include push-ups, chest presses, dumbbell flyes, and resistance band exercises. Each exercise will be explained in detail, highlighting the muscle groups being engaged and the proper form to maximize effectiveness and safety.

Incorporating Resistance Training for Bust Firmness

Resistance training is a powerful tool for enhancing bust elasticity. We'll discuss the benefits of using weights or resistance bands to challenge the muscles and stimulate growth. By progressively increasing resistance over time, you can gradually enhance the strength and tone of the pectoral muscles, leading to improved bust support and appearance.

Yoga and Stretching for Bust Flexibility

Flexibility is an integral aspect of bust health and posture. We'll explore how yoga and stretching can promote flexibility and mobility in the chest, shoulders, and back – areas that contribute to overall bust appearance. Gentle stretches and yoga poses can help prevent muscle tightness and improve circulation, supporting bust elasticity.

Creating a Bust-Focused Exercise Routine

Building a well-rounded exercise routine that targets bust muscles requires careful planning. We'll discuss how to structure your workouts to incorporate bust-focused exercises alongside full-body and cardiovascular workouts. A balanced approach ensures that you address all aspects of fitness while prioritizing bust health.

Progressive Training and Monitoring Results

Like any fitness endeavor, consistency and progression are key. We'll delve into the concept of progressive overload, where you gradually increase the intensity of your exercises over time. Additionally, we'll explore methods for tracking your progress and monitoring changes in bust appearance, muscle tone, and overall strength.

Customizing Your Exercise Plan

Every individual is unique, and exercise preferences vary. We'll provide guidance on tailoring your bust-focused exercise routine to your fitness level, goals, and preferences. Whether you're a beginner or have prior experience, customization ensures that your exercise plan aligns with your personal journey toward enhanced bust elasticity.

Safety Considerations and Precautions

Exercise safety is paramount. We'll discuss common safety considerations and precautions to take while engaging in bust-focused exercises. Proper form, appropriate warm-up routines, and listening to your body are essential components of a safe and effective exercise regimen.

As you delve into bust-focused exercises, you'll discover a range of options to strengthen and support the muscles that contribute to bust elasticity. By incorporating these exercises into your fitness routine and embracing a holistic approach to health, you can embark on a journey to enhance the strength, appearance, and vitality of your bust.

Chapter 5: Maintaining Proper Posture

In this chapter, we explore the significant role that proper posture plays in promoting bust health, appearance, and overall well-being. While often overlooked, maintaining good posture is essential for preventing strain on the muscles and ligaments that support the bust. By understanding the importance of posture and incorporating mindful practices into your daily routine, you can positively impact your bust's elasticity and contribute to a confident and healthy physique.

The Importance of Posture for Bust Appearance

Proper posture not only affects your overall appearance but also has a direct impact on how your bust is perceived. We'll delve into how slouching or poor posture can lead to a less-than-ideal bust presentation, potentially contributing to sagging and discomfort. By maintaining an upright posture, you create a more flattering and supportive environment for the bust.

Exercises to Improve Posture and Bust Alignment
We'll explore a range of exercises and stretches designed to enhance your posture and align the

spine. These exercises may include shoulder blade squeezes, chin tucks, and wall angels. By engaging the muscles that support proper posture, you can counteract the effects of prolonged sitting and other common habits that contribute to poor posture.

Ergonomics and Bust Health in Everyday Activities

Beyond exercise, the way you carry out daily activities – such as sitting, standing, and working – significantly impacts your posture and bust health. We'll discuss the principles of ergonomic design and how to create supportive environments that encourage proper posture. By making small adjustments to your workspace and habits, you can maintain a posture-friendly lifestyle.

Posture and Confidence

Proper posture not only affects physical health but also influences your mental and emotional state. We'll explore the connection between posture and confidence, discussing how standing tall and owning your space can boost self-esteem and body image. By recognizing the link between posture and emotional well-being, you can cultivate a positive self-perception that radiates from within.

Incorporating Posture Practices into Daily Life

We'll provide practical tips and strategies for incorporating posture-improving practices into your daily routine. From mindful posture checks to creating reminders for yourself, these simple yet effective strategies can help you build lasting habits that support bust health.

Posture and Age-Related Changes

As we age, maintaining proper posture becomes increasingly important for preserving bust elasticity and preventing sagging. We'll discuss how age-related changes in posture and muscle tone can impact the bust area and share strategies to counteract these effects. By embracing posture-enhancing practices, you can navigate the natural aging process with grace and confidence.

Holistic Wellness and Posture

Proper posture is an integral aspect of holistic wellness. We'll explore how posture aligns with other elements of well-being, such as physical fitness, emotional health, and self-care. By recognizing the interconnectedness of these aspects, you can embrace a comprehensive approach to wellness that supports your bust's elasticity and overall vitality.

Long-Term Posture Maintenance

Maintaining proper posture is a lifelong commitment. We'll discuss strategies for sustaining good posture as you navigate different life stages, from adolescence to adulthood and beyond. By consistently practicing posture-improving techniques, you can ensure the ongoing health and appearance of your bust.

As you delve into the world of proper posture, you'll gain valuable insights into how your body's alignment affects your bust health and overall well-being. By incorporating posture-enhancing practices into your daily life, you can create a supportive foundation that contributes to the long-term elasticity and vibrancy of your bust.

Chapter 6: Skincare and Bust Elasticity

In this chapter, we shift our focus to the external care of the bust area through skincare practices that contribute to maintaining its elasticity, suppleness, and overall health. Just as we prioritize skincare for our face and body, the skin on the bust requires attention and care to ensure its vitality and support its underlying structures. By understanding the unique needs of the bust area and adopting effective skincare routines, you can nurture your skin and enhance its appearance.

Understanding Bust Skin Anatomy

Before delving into skincare practices, it's essential to grasp the anatomical features of the bust skin. We'll explore the structure and characteristics of bust skin, including its thickness, elasticity, and susceptibility to stretch marks. Understanding these factors will provide insight into the specific skincare needs of the bust area.

Choosing the Right Skincare Products

We'll discuss the importance of selecting appropriate skincare products that cater to the delicate skin of the bust. From cleansers and moisturizers to serums and sunscreens, we'll explore ingredients and formulations that promote skin health and elasticity. By making informed choices, you can create a skincare regimen that addresses the unique needs of the bust.

Massage Techniques to Enhance Bust Elasticity

Regular massage can play a significant role in maintaining skin elasticity and improving blood circulation in the bust area. We'll delve into massage techniques that stimulate collagen production, increase lymphatic drainage, and promote overall skin health. By incorporating these techniques into your routine, you can contribute to the suppleness and vitality of the bust.

Prevention of Stretch Marks and Skin Laxity

Stretch marks and skin laxity are common concerns in the bust area. We'll explore strategies for preventing and minimizing the appearance of stretch marks, as well as techniques to improve skin firmness. By adopting a proactive approach to skincare, you can work to reduce the impact of factors that contribute to skin changes over time.

Hydration and Moisturization for Bust Skin

Hydrated skin is more resilient and elastic. We'll discuss the role of proper hydration and moisturization in maintaining the health and appearance of the bust. Understanding how to effectively moisturize and lock in hydration can contribute to a more youthful and vibrant bust complexion.

Sun Protection and UV Exposure

Sun damage can affect the elasticity and health of the skin. We'll explore the importance of sun protection in the bust area and discuss strategies for safeguarding your skin from harmful UV rays. By adopting sun-safe practices, you can help prevent premature aging and maintain the integrity of your bust skin.

Skincare Rituals for Bust Health

We'll provide guidance on creating a comprehensive skincare ritual that incorporates cleansing, exfoliation, massage, moisturization, and sun protection. A consistent skincare routine tailored to the unique needs of the bust area can contribute to its long-term health and vitality.

Natural Remedies and DIY Skincare

For those interested in natural approaches, we'll explore DIY skincare recipes and remedies that can be easily prepared at home. These natural treatments can complement your skincare routine and provide additional nourishment to the bust skin.

Sustaining Bust Skin Health

Lastly, we'll discuss strategies for sustaining the benefits of your skincare efforts over time. By consistently practicing effective skincare and adapting your routine as needed, you can support the elasticity and appearance of your bust skin throughout different life stages.

As you explore the world of skincare for bust health, you'll gain insights into how external care can contribute to the overall elasticity and vitality of the bust area. By incorporating these skincare practices into your daily routine, you can nurture your skin and contribute to the long-term health and appearance of your bust.

Chapter 7: Lifestyle Factors and Bust lasticity

In this chapter, we examine how various lifestyle factors influence bust elasticity and overall breast health. Our daily habits, choices, and behaviors play a significant role in shaping the condition of our bodies, including the bust area. By understanding the impact of lifestyle factors and making conscious decisions, you can proactively contribute to the long-term health, appearance, and resilience of your bust.

Nutrition's Role in Lifestyle

We revisit the pivotal role of nutrition and its direct influence on bust health. From the foods we consume to the timing of our meals, we'll explore how dietary choices and habits impact the quality of breast tissue, collagen production, and overall elasticity. By adopting a balanced and nutrient-rich diet, you can align your eating habits with your aspirations for optimal bust health.

Hydration and Lifestyle

Adequate hydration is crucial not only for overall health but also for maintaining skin elasticity and preventing dryness. We'll discuss how lifestyle factors such as fluid intake, caffeine consumption, and alcohol use can affect hydration levels and consequently influence the health of the bust skin and underlying tissues. By prioritizing hydration, you support the vibrancy and elasticity of your bust.

Physical Activity and Bust Health

Regular physical activity is a cornerstone of a healthy lifestyle and has a direct impact on bust elasticity. We'll explore how a sedentary lifestyle and lack of exercise can contribute to weakened muscles, poor circulation, and compromised posture – factors that affect bust appearance and support. By incorporating movement and exercise into your daily routine, you can enhance muscle tone, circulation, and overall bust health.

Sleep Quality and Bust Elasticity

Sleep is a restorative process that affects various aspects of health, including the skin's elasticity and appearance. We'll discuss the relationship between sleep quality, cellular regeneration, and the maintenance of healthy breast tissue. Strategies for improving sleep hygiene and prioritizing restful sleep can contribute to the long-term health of your bust.

Stress Management and Emotional Well-Being

Chronic stress can have a profound impact on the body, including the bust area. We'll delve into the effects of stress hormones on collagen and elastin production, as well as the potential for stress-induced habits like poor posture. Strategies for managing stress, such as mindfulness, relaxation techniques, and self-care practices, can positively influence bust elasticity and overall well-being.

Tobacco and Alcohol Consumption

The choices we make regarding tobacco and alcohol consumption can significantly affect skin health and elasticity. We'll explore how smoking and excessive alcohol use can deplete the skin of essential nutrients, impair circulation, and accelerate aging. Understanding the impact of these substances on bust health can motivate you to make healthier choices that support elasticity.

Weight Management and Bust Appearance

Maintaining a healthy weight is essential for overall health and has implications for bust appearance. We'll discuss how fluctuations in weight, both weight gain and weight loss, can impact the skin's elasticity and the structural integrity of breast tissue. By adopting a balanced approach to weight management, you can promote the long-term health and resilience of your bust.

Environmental Factors and Lifestyle Choices

External environmental factors, such as sun exposure and pollution, can influence the skin's health and elasticity. We'll explore how lifestyle choices, such as wearing sunscreen and minimizing exposure to pollutants, can protect the bust area from premature aging and maintain its vitality.

Sustainable Lifestyle Habits for Bust Elasticity

Incorporating sustainable lifestyle habits is essential for maintaining the benefits over time. We'll discuss strategies for creating lasting changes that align with your values and goals. By adopting habits that support bust elasticity and overall health, you can contribute to the long-term well-being of your bust.

As you navigate the intricate web of lifestyle factors, you'll gain a deeper understanding of how your daily choices impact the elasticity and appearance of your bust. By making informed decisions and embracing a holistic approach to well-being, you can create a lifestyle that nurtures your bust's health and vitality for years to come.

Chapter 8: Bras and Bust Support

In this chapter, we delve into the critical role that bras play in providing proper support, comfort, and maintaining the elasticity of the bust. Wearing the right type of bra can significantly impact breast health, appearance, and overall well-being. By understanding the importance of bra selection, fit, and care, you can ensure that your bust receives the necessary support to maintain its elasticity and vitality.

The Importance of Proper Bust Support

We begin by exploring why proper bust support is essential for maintaining the health and elasticity of breast tissue. We'll discuss how bras help distribute weight, reduce strain, and prevent sagging – factors that directly influence bust appearance and comfort. By recognizing the significance of adequate support, you can make informed decisions when choosing bras.

Bra Types and Their Impact on Bust Health

We'll delve into different types of bras, such as sports bras, underwire bras, and wireless bras, and discuss their specific benefits and considerations for bust support. We'll explore how each type of bra affects circulation, movement, and overall breast health. By understanding the characteristics of various bras, you can choose the most suitable options for your needs.

Bra Fitting and Bust Elasticity

A well-fitting bra is crucial for providing optimal support and preventing unnecessary strain on breast tissue. We'll guide you through the process of finding the right bra size, including measuring techniques and signs of an ill-fitting bra. By wearing bras that fit correctly, you can minimize the risk of discomfort and potential negative effects on bust elasticity.

The Impact of Sports Bras on Bust Elasticity

Exercise and physical activity require specialized support to maintain bust health during movement. We'll discuss the importance of sports bras in preventing excessive bouncing and stress on breast tissue. We'll explore how sports bras contribute to maintaining bust elasticity during workouts and activities.

Bras and Posture Improvement

Properly fitting bras can also have a positive impact on posture. We'll discuss how bras with adequate support can promote better posture by distributing weight and encouraging an upright stance. Improved posture can contribute to bust health, overall body alignment, and appearance.

Choosing Bras for Different Occasions

Different activities and outfits call for different types of bras. We'll provide guidance on selecting appropriate bras for various occasions, from everyday wear to special events, and discuss how these choices can influence bust health and comfort. By having a range of bras that cater to different needs, you can ensure consistent support and comfort.

Bra Care and Longevity

Maintaining the quality and functionality of your bras is essential for ongoing bust support. We'll share tips for proper bra care, including washing, storage, and lifespan considerations. By taking care of your bras, you can ensure they provide reliable support and contribute to the long-term elasticity of your bust.

Embracing Bra-Free Time

While proper bra support is crucial, there are instances where going bra-free can be beneficial. We'll explore the importance of allowing your bust to breathe and the potential benefits of going bra-free for short periods. By finding a balance between supportive bra wear and bra-free time, you can contribute to bust health and comfort.

Lifestyle and Bra Choices

We'll discuss how lifestyle factors, such as activity level, wardrobe preferences, and comfort, should guide your bra choices. By aligning your bra selection with your daily activities and preferences, you can ensure consistent and appropriate support that promotes bust elasticity and overall well-being.

As you navigate the world of bras and bust support, you'll gain a deeper understanding of how proper bra choices and fit contribute to the elasticity, comfort, and appearance of your bust. By selecting bras that offer the right support for your needs and taking care of them, you can maintain the health and vitality of your bust for years to come.

Chapter 9: Natural Remedies and Herbal Supplements

In this chapter, we explore the realm of natural remedies and herbal supplements as potential contributors to bust health and elasticity. Natural remedies and herbs have been used for centuries to promote well-being and address various health concerns. We'll examine how certain plants, herbs, and natural substances are thought to influence bust health and offer insights into their potential benefits and considerations.

Exploring Herbal Tradition

We begin by delving into the historical and cultural use of herbs and natural remedies for health and beauty. We'll discuss how various cultures have embraced herbal traditions and integrated them into daily practices. Understanding the roots of herbalism provides context for exploring their potential role in maintaining bust health.

Herbs and Plants for Bust Health

We'll explore specific herbs and plants that are traditionally associated with supporting breast health and elasticity. Examples may include fenugreek, fennel, red clover, wild yam, and saw palmetto. We'll discuss the potential mechanisms through which these herbs may impact hormonal balance, collagen production, and overall breast well-being.

Potential Benefits of Herbal Supplements

Certain herbal supplements are believed to contribute to breast health and elasticity through their unique properties. We'll discuss how these supplements may interact with the body and influence factors such as hormone regulation, circulation, and tissue support. By understanding the potential benefits, you can make informed decisions about incorporating herbal supplements into your routine.

Considerations and Safety

While herbal remedies offer potential benefits, it's important to approach them with caution and awareness. We'll discuss considerations such as dosage, interactions with medications, and potential side effects. Consulting with a healthcare professional before introducing herbal supplements is advisable to ensure their compatibility with your individual health profile.

Nutritional Support from Herbal Teas

Herbal teas can provide a soothing and nourishing way to incorporate herbs into your routine. We'll explore herbal teas that are known for their potential benefits to breast health, such as dandelion root, red raspberry leaf, and fenugreek tea. These teas offer an enjoyable and hydrating means of embracing herbal support.

DIY Herbal Remedies and Topical Applications

We'll provide guidance on preparing and using DIY herbal remedies, such as herbal-infused oils or creams, for external application to the bust area. These topical treatments can provide nourishment and hydration to the skin, contributing to its elasticity and overall health.

Balancing Herbal Approaches with Other Strategies

Herbal remedies can complement other lifestyle factors we've explored in previous chapters. We'll discuss how herbal support can align with practices such as skincare, exercise, and proper posture. By integrating herbal remedies into a comprehensive approach, you can create a well-rounded regimen that addresses various aspects of bust health.

Embracing Holistic Wellness

Ultimately, the integration of natural remedies and herbal supplements aligns with a holistic approach to well-being. We'll discuss how the holistic perspective recognizes the interconnectedness of physical, emotional, and spiritual aspects of health. By embracing holistic wellness, you can create a harmonious and balanced environment that supports your bust's elasticity and vitality.

Consultation with Healthcare Professionals

Throughout this chapter, we emphasize the importance of consulting with healthcare professionals before introducing herbal supplements or remedies into your routine. Their expertise can help you make informed choices that align with your individual health needs and goals.

As you explore the world of natural remedies and herbal supplements, you'll gain insights into how these traditional practices can potentially contribute to bust health and elasticity. By approaching herbal support with mindfulness, consideration, and a holistic perspective, you can create a well-rounded approach to maintaining the health and vitality of your bust.

Chapter 10: Surgical and Medical Interventions

In this chapter, we delve into the realm of surgical and medical interventions as options for addressing bust health, appearance, and elasticity. While the previous chapters have focused on natural and lifestyle approaches, it's important to acknowledge that medical interventions can also play a role in enhancing bust elasticity. We'll explore various surgical and medical options, their potential benefits, considerations, and the importance of informed decision-making.

Introduction to Surgical and Medical Interventions

We begin by providing an overview of the surgical and medical interventions available for individuals seeking to enhance or address bust health and elasticity. From surgical procedures to minimally invasive treatments, we'll discuss the range of options available and their potential outcomes.

Breast Augmentation and Reduction Surgery

We'll explore breast augmentation surgery, which involves enhancing breast size using implants or fat transfer. Additionally, we'll discuss breast reduction surgery, which is aimed at reducing breast size and improving comfort. Both procedures can have an impact on bust appearance and the distribution of breast tissue.

Breast Lift Surgery (Mastopexy)

Breast lift surgery, also known as mastopexy, is a procedure designed to lift and reshape sagging breasts. We'll discuss how this surgery can address issues related to bust elasticity, particularly in cases where sagging has occurred due to factors such as pregnancy, weight loss, or aging.

Lipofilling and Fat Transfer

Lipofilling, or fat transfer, involves using a person's own fat cells to enhance the size and shape of the breasts. We'll explore how this minimally invasive procedure can impact bust appearance and potentially contribute to bust elasticity.

Non-Surgical Treatments and Procedures

Beyond surgical options, we'll discuss non-surgical treatments and procedures that can address bust health and elasticity. These may include ultrasound therapy, radiofrequency treatments, and laser therapies. We'll explore their potential benefits, mechanisms, and considerations.

Patient Considerations and Decision-Making

Making the decision to undergo a surgical or medical intervention is a significant choice. We'll discuss important considerations such as candidacy, risks, benefits, recovery, and expected outcomes. We'll emphasize the importance of thorough research, consultation with qualified professionals, and informed decision-making.

Holistic Approach to Interventions

We'll explore how surgical and medical interventions can be integrated into a holistic approach to well-being. While these interventions offer specific benefits, they are most effective when combined with other factors such as lifestyle, skincare, and exercise. A comprehensive approach supports long-term bust health and vitality.

Consultation with Healthcare Professionals

Throughout this chapter, we emphasize the critical importance of consulting with qualified healthcare professionals. Whether considering surgery or non-surgical treatments, a thorough consultation ensures that you receive accurate information, personalized recommendations, and a clear understanding of the options available.

Personalized Approach and Empowerment

Every individual's journey is unique, and there is no one-size-fits-all solution. We encourage you to consider your personal goals, preferences, and health circumstances when exploring surgical and medical interventions. By taking an empowered and informed approach, you can make choices that align with your aspirations for bust health and elasticity.

As you explore the world of surgical and medical interventions, you'll gain insights into the potential options available to enhance bust health and elasticity. By approaching these interventions with careful consideration, consultation, and a holistic perspective, you can make choices that support your individual goals and contribute to your overall well-being.

Chapter 11: Embracing Body Positivity and Self-Care

In this final chapter, we shift our focus towards the emotional and psychological aspects of bust health and elasticity. Embracing body positivity and practicing self-care are fundamental components of overall well-being that directly impact how you perceive, care for, and nurture your body. By fostering a positive relationship with your body and prioritizing self-care practices, you can enhance your bust's elasticity and contribute to a healthier, more fulfilling life.

Understanding Body Positivity

We begin by exploring the concept of body positivity – a movement that promotes self-acceptance, self-love, and appreciation for all body types. We'll discuss the importance of recognizing and challenging societal beauty standards that can influence body image. Embracing body positivity encourages you to celebrate your body's uniqueness and cultivate a positive self-perception.

Body Image and Bust Health

We'll delve into how body image influences not only your emotional well-being but also your physical health, including bust elasticity. Negative body image and self-criticism can contribute to stress, which in turn may impact hormonal balance and overall health. By fostering a positive body image, you create a supportive environment for bust health and overall vitality.

The Role of Self-Care in Bust Health

Self-care encompasses a range of practices that prioritize your mental, emotional, and physical well-being. We'll explore how self-care rituals, such as mindfulness, meditation, journaling, and spending time in nature, can positively impact stress levels, hormone regulation, and ultimately, bust health. Engaging in regular self-care activities supports overall body wellness, including the bust area.

Cultivating Self-Love and Confidence

We'll discuss strategies for cultivating self-love and confidence, which are essential components of a healthy body image. Embracing self-affirmations, gratitude, and positive self-talk can contribute to a sense of empowerment and appreciation for your body's resilience and uniqueness.

Overcoming Negative Thought Patterns

Negative thought patterns can undermine body positivity and self-care efforts. We'll explore techniques for challenging and reframing negative thoughts related to body image. By adopting a more compassionate and realistic perspective, you can release self-criticism and create a more nurturing mindset.

Mindful Eating and Intuitive Nourishment

Mindful eating and intuitive nourishment involve paying attention to your body's cues and responding to its needs with kindness. We'll discuss how these practices can support a healthy relationship with food and contribute to hormonal balance, digestion, and overall well-being, including bust health.

Celebrating Your Body's Journey

Embracing body positivity involves recognizing and celebrating your body's journey and the experiences that have shaped it. We'll discuss the significance of acknowledging the changes your body has gone through and appreciating its resilience. This perspective contributes to a sense of acceptance and gratitude for your body, including your bust.

Holistic Wellness and Emotional Health

Finally, we'll explore the interconnectedness of emotional health and physical well-being. By prioritizing emotional wellness, you create an environment that positively impacts hormonal balance, stress levels, and overall health. A holistic approach that nurtures both your emotional and physical needs contributes to the elasticity and vitality of your bust.

Embracing Your Unique Journey

In this chapter, we encourage you to embrace your unique journey towards bust health and elasticity. By practicing body positivity, self-care, and cultivating a loving relationship with your body, you can create a harmonious and nurturing environment that supports your well-being in all aspects of life.

As you explore the concepts of body positivity and self-care, you'll gain valuable insights into how these practices contribute to bust health, elasticity, and overall well-being. By fostering a positive and compassionate relationship with your body, you embark on a journey of empowerment, self-discovery, and lasting vitality.

Chapter 12: Maintenance and Long-Term Strategies

In the final chapter of the book, we focus on maintenance and long-term strategies for preserving the elasticity, health, and appearance of your bust. Just as consistent care is essential for overall well-being, ongoing attention to bust health is crucial for maintaining the results you've achieved and promoting lasting vitality. We'll discuss a range of practices, habits, and considerations that will help you sustain your efforts and continue to enjoy the benefits of enhanced bust elasticity.

Creating a Sustainable Routine

We begin by emphasizing the importance of creating a sustainable routine that aligns with your lifestyle and goals. We'll explore how consistency in skincare, exercise, nutrition, and other aspects of bust care contributes to long-term results. Building habits that you can maintain over time ensures that your efforts to enhance bust elasticity remain effective.

Regular Bust Self-Assessment

We'll discuss the value of regular self-assessment as a means of tracking changes in bust health and appearance. By periodically evaluating your bust's elasticity, skin texture, and overall well-being, you can identify any shifts or concerns and adjust your routine accordingly. Self-assessment empowers you to proactively address any changes and continue to nurture your bust's health.

Adapting to Life Stages

Throughout life, your body undergoes various changes that can impact bust health. We'll explore how different life stages, such as puberty, pregnancy, menopause, and aging, can influence bust elasticity and appearance. We'll discuss strategies for adapting your care routine to accommodate these transitions and maintain bust health through each stage.

Incorporating Learnings from Earlier Chapters

We'll revisit key takeaways from earlier chapters of the book and discuss how to integrate them into your ongoing maintenance routine. Whether it's skincare practices, exercise routines, posture improvement, or emotional well-being, each aspect contributes to the overall health and elasticity of your bust.

Consulting Professionals as Needed

Regular consultations with healthcare professionals, such as dermatologists, fitness experts, nutritionists, and gynecologists, remain valuable throughout your journey. We'll discuss how seeking expert guidance and assessments can help you fine-tune your approach and ensure that you're on track for maintaining bust health and elasticity.

Long-Term Mindset and Patience

Maintaining bust health and elasticity is a long-term commitment that requires patience and a positive mindset. We'll explore how cultivating a long-term perspective and embracing the journey – with its ups and downs – contributes to sustainable results. By recognizing that changes take time, you can stay motivated and focused on your goals.

Celebrating Progress and Self-Care Rituals

We'll discuss the importance of celebrating your progress and milestones along the way. Self-care rituals, whether it's a relaxing bath, a special treat, or a moment of mindfulness, contribute to emotional well-being and foster a sense of accomplishment. Celebrating your efforts enhances your motivation to continue caring for your bust's health.

Supportive Community and Accountability

Having a supportive community or partner can bolster your commitment to maintaining bust health. We'll explore how sharing your goals, progress, and challenges with others can provide accountability, encouragement, and a sense of camaraderie. Connecting with like-minded individuals can make the journey more enjoyable and rewarding.

Lifelong Journey of Self-Care

Lastly, we'll reflect on how maintaining bust health and elasticity is part of a larger journey of self-care and well-being. By embracing a holistic approach to health, you invest in your overall vitality and quality of life. Your commitment to self-care and maintenance is an ongoing expression of self-love and empowerment.

As you embark on the path of maintenance and long-term strategies, you'll gain a deeper understanding of how consistent care, adaptation, and a positive mindset contribute to the lasting health and elasticity of your bust. By embracing this journey as an integral part of your life, you can continue to enjoy the benefits of enhanced bust vitality and overall well-being.